P9-DEY-328

FOREWORD

Welcome to the fourth – and likely final – installment of Unreported Truths.

If I had time, I would write more booklets: about flaws in PCR testing and how they have made the pandemic appear worse than it is; about the harm done by school closures and the way teachers' unions have used Covid to hurt children; about the murky origins of the Sars-Cov-2 virus.

But I don't have time. I have a book called PANDEMIA to write, and it is due all-too-soon. And we seem to be leaving the crisis phase of the pandemic behind. The winter spike has come and gone in the United States and almost everywhere else. With luck, we will have no big spring or summer spike, and even the most panicked among us will begin to resume their lives.

I started writing the Unreported Truths booklets last May. I wanted to speak out about the unfolding crisis I saw – a crisis created less by the pandemic than by our panicked response to it. They are simple and urgent, black and white, no charts or graphs. They are filled with facts, not feelings. They are informative, not writerly. They are, to use an insult that seemed fashionable among teenagers for a while, basic.

Now I need to step back and write something a little less basic. We all need to step back, even if doing so is difficult in an age of real-time death counts on CNN and 280-character bulletins on Twitter. Over the last year, governments around the world have scissored our personal freedoms in a way no one would have expected before March 2020. They have locked us down and made us wear masks and closed our schools with almost no oversight or pushback, to combat a virus that kills 1 or 2 of every 1,000 people it infects worldwide.

We need to think about whether what we have done makes any sense, and how to make sure we don't make the same mistakes next time. Because there will be a next time.

So I will be laying off Twitter a bit (I hope) and devoting my energies to PANDEMIA.

But first I needed to write this Unreported Truths, about vaccines.

The media and public health experts have engaged in dangerous groupthink since last March. But their unwillingness to examine hard data or ask tough questions has reached new heights with vaccines.

As you'll see when you read this booklet, I am far from an anti-vaxxer. But I believe we should have looked harder at the pros and cons of these new vaccines, especially the ones from Moderna and Pfizer, before we decided to push them on eight billion people around the world.

We have surprisingly little information about these vaccines. After all, none of them even existed at the start of 2020. Yet somehow that mystery paradoxically has worked almost to their benefit. Regulators and governments and journalists have treated them as magic potions that will fix a year of mistakes, rather than what they are: incredibly complex technology that carries real risks. I hope this booklet, without being alarmist, will give you a better idea of what those risks are, and how much we *don't* know.

Magic potions belong in fairy tales, not medicine.

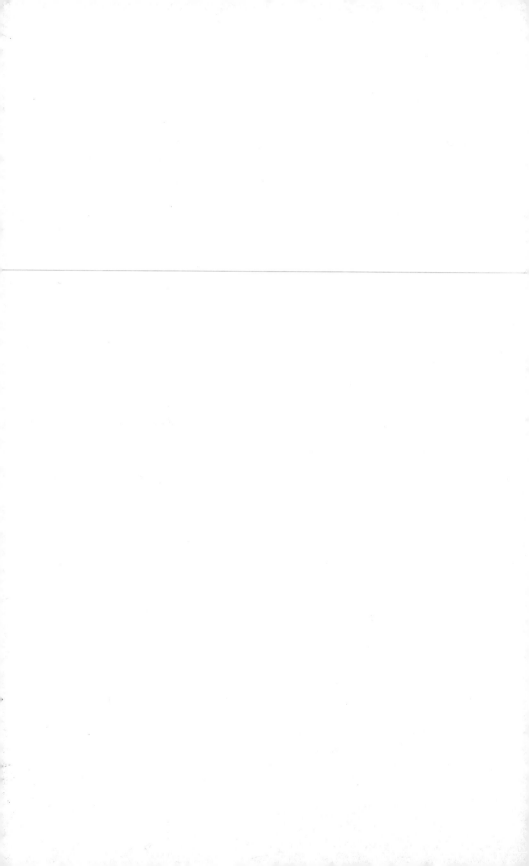

INTRODUCTION

At 6:45 a.m. on November 9, 2020, the United States woke to stunning news:

Testing of a new coronavirus vaccine had shown hugely positive results. The vaccine, from the American drug maker Pfizer and its German partner BioNTech, nearly ended infections in the 20,000 people who received it, Pfizer said.

"Pfizer's Covid-19 Vaccine Proves 90% Effective in Latest Trials," The Wall Street Journal reported. The Journal said the finding was "much better than anticipated" and "marks a milestone in the hunt for shots that can stop the pandemic."

Days later, the news turned even better. Updated data showed Pfizer's vaccine and a similar shot from a Massachusetts biotechnology company called Moderna cut the risk of infection by up to 95 percent.

Further, both companies said their products looked safe. "No serious safety concerns have been observed," Pfizer reported. Moderna said its vaccine "was generally well tolerated."

After nine grim Covid-filled months, the vaccine findings looked like a giant victory for science and medicine. They offered a path back to normal life. They'd also come much faster than expected. When Covid first emerged from China in early 2020, vaccine experts had predicted shots against Sars-Cov-2 would not be ready until late 2021 at the earliest.

The experts had also warned the vaccines might offer only modest protection, preventing infections in half or two-thirds of the people who received them. In Senate testimony in September, Dr. Robert Redfield, the head of the Centers for Disease Control, even said vaccines might not work as well as masks.

(https://www.cnbc.com/2020/09/16/cdc-director-says-face-masks-may-provide-more-protection-than-coronavirus-vaccine-.html)

Instead, scientists around the world had come together in a government-academic-private partnership to offer protection to a desperate planet.

"These are obviously very exciting results," Dr. Anthony Fauci told CNN after Moderna released its data on Nov. 16. "It's just as good as it gets." (https://www.cnn.com/2020/11/16/health/moderna-vaccine-results-coronavirus/index.html)

Debates about which lucky people should have first chance at the vaccines began immediately. The stocks of Moderna and BioNTech, which had jumped during 2020 alongside rising hopes for the vaccines, soared even further after the announcements.

Company executives and scientists basked in praise. A Nov. 10 article in The Guardian, a British newspaper, explained how a husband and wife in Germany – Dr. Ugur Sahin and Dr. Ozlem Tureci, both physicians, both the children of Turkish migrants – had founded BioNTech.

"They are the 'dream team' scientist couple who came up with a big idea that could protect humanity from a virus that has killed more than a million people," the Guardian wrote. "The couple married in 2002, interrupting their research only briefly to slip out of their lab coats and dash to the registry office on their wedding day."

(https://www.theguardian.com/world/2020/nov/10/ugur-sahin-and-ozlem-tureci-german-dream-team-behind-vaccine)

A Nov. 30 article about Moderna in The New York Times was equally glowing. It ended with the moment that chief executive Stephane Bancel received the results in a conference call on Sun., Nov. 15, and raced to let his family know:

> He ducked out into the hallway to tell his wife. His 18-year old daughter raced down from the second floor. His 16-year-old flew up the basement stairs.
>
> "The four of us were crying," he said.

(https://www.nytimes.com/2020/11/21/us/politics/coronavirus-vaccine.html)

A Hollywood ending for the ages. The tale of the Pfizer and Moderna vaccines seemed almost too good to be true.

And it is.

I am not a vaccine denier.

Let's get that nonsense out of the way first.

I was vaccinated as a kid. Our children have gotten their shots on schedule, with no ill effects aside from a few tears. I don't personally know anyone who has ever suffered any negative effects from childhood vaccinations.

I acknowledge I have not studied the risks of childhood vaccines in any detail. I know they can very occasionally cause serious reactions. But I suspect rising reported rates of autism – sometimes blamed on vaccines – are more likely tied to changes in the way we label children with developmental problems.

Autism diagnoses have soared in recent decades. But diagnoses of mental retardation, which parents consider more stigmatizing, have plunged. The switch suggests that some children who once might have been categorized as having retardation are now called autistic.

I even think public schools should make some vaccines mandatory, such as for measles and polio. Those viruses carry a small but real risk of death for kids. They can be prevented with vaccines that rely on simple and well-understood mechanisms of action. Generations of vaccinations have proven the risk is very low.

So. I am not an anti-vaxxer. (I write this knowing that I have disappointed many of my natural allies on this issue.)

But the term "anti-vaxxer" is itself problematic. Pointing out that thalidomide can cause birth defects wouldn't make me an "anti-mediciner." Some drugs, like HIV treatments, are lifesavers. Others may not work at all, or have side effects that outweigh their benefits. We depend on painstaking research and clinical trials to reveal their pluses and minuses. We ask regulators to keep the risky ones off the market. That's true of vaccines too. But the bar should be even higher for vaccines, which are given to healthy people rather than those who are already ill.

I wish we could trust the pharmaceutical industry to be honest about these new vaccines. But I am a cynic, especially about Big Pharma. The years I spent covering it for The New York Times taught me the games drug companies play in their research and marketing. They overestimate how well their medicines work and underestimate side effects.

Pharma's tactics can be dangerous even for well-understood medicines with long histories. In this case, though, the stakes are far higher. The Pfizer and Moderna vaccines are nearly identical, and both work far differently than earlier types of vaccines. (I will generally refer to the Pfizer/BioNTech vaccine as "Pfizer," even though the companies are equal partners.) Some scientists question whether they should be called vaccines at all, or whether they are more properly classified as gene therapies, since they temporarily insert foreign genetic material called mRNA into our cells.

Until December, drug regulators had *never* allowed the sale of any vaccine or drug based on mRNA technology. Moderna had stumbled for years as it tried to create similar vaccines for influenza and other viruses. The company was nowhere near gaining approval despite burning through billions of dollars on research. No surprise, as drug development is normally a glacial process – understandably, given the risks.

Not this time, though. Regulators okayed both Covid vaccines in a matter of *weeks* after Pfizer and Moderna announced their clinical trial results. Leaked emails from European drug regulators show that they and their American counterparts were under extraordinary political pressure to approve the mRNA vaccines even without conducting a full scientific and medical review.

An important side note: I am focusing almost exclusively on the mRNA vaccines in this booklet, because far more Americans have received them than the Johnson & Johnson vaccine, which is the only other authorized vaccine in the United States. In addition, the J&J vaccine had fewer side effects in clinical trials. European regulators have approved a fourth major vaccine, from AstraZeneca. But Germany and other countries have now suspended its use because of concerns about side effects. I will discuss the AstraZeneca vaccine briefly later, because the issues the suspension raises are relevant to the mRNA vaccines. But since it is not currently sold in the United States, I am not going to focus on it.

And as soon as the vaccine authorizations began – in Britain on Dec. 2, in the United States on Dec. 11, in Europe on Dec. 21 – government agencies like the Centers for Disease Control campaigned to encourage reluctant people to get shots. Scientists and politicians have even discussed making vaccinations mandatory for healthy adults, an unprecedented step. Companies like United Airlines have said they want to force employees to be vaccinated. Schools are warning parents of mandatory vaccinations as soon as regulators approve Covid shots for kids.

Well over 100 million people have already received the Pfizer and Moderna shots, and millions more are getting them every day. The final total may top one billion worldwide. To prepare, wealthy countries have ordered billions of Covid vaccine doses. The United States, the United Kingdom, and the European Union have bought 3.2 billion doses, enough to vaccinate their entire populations twice over even at two shots per person. Canada has gone even further, ordering almost 10 doses for every citizen.

(https://www.theguardian.com/world/2021/jan/29/canada-and-uk-among-countries-with-most-vaccine-doses-ordered-per-person)

Yet if something goes wrong with the vaccines, the companies that make them face no legal risk.

The United States and other countries have offered Covid vaccine manufacturers immunity from vaccine-related lawsuits. In general, after-the-fact legal action is a crude and expensive tool to keep companies from taking chances with public health. Regulation is preferable. But where regulators have greased the skids, potential liability helps hold companies accountable. Removing it also means companies will never have to turn their internal documents over to plaintiffs' lawyers or the media.

Given the stakes, journalists should look hard at what we know about these treatments. Instead, they have pretended the science around these new vaccines is more settled than it is. They have ignored serious problems in the clinical trial data and the real-world experience of countries like Israel and Britain since the vaccines were authorized for use in December.

Instead of skepticism, major media outlets have pushed the vaccines even harder than lockdowns and masks – pretending they are a risk-free choice, just as they did with those "non-pharmaceutical interventions."

It is time – past time – to stop cheerleading and start asking the questions we should have posed before we ever allowed these vaccines to be sold.

1

If you've read earlier sections of Unreported Truths, you know I believe cloth and surgical masks do not protect their wearers from Covid. Anyone who says otherwise is ignoring decades of research. In November, a study of thousands of people in Denmark proved that masks did not reduce coronavirus infections in people who wore them.

Similarly, I think lockdowns generally do more harm than good.

Let me be clear: The situation with vaccines is different.

We have evidence that the mRNA and other vaccines *do* work, at least to reduce mild or moderate infections.

How? Pfizer and other vaccine makers all tested their shots in double-blinded, randomized clinical trials. Those trials are the best way to judge whether a drug or vaccine works.

To run the trials, the companies recruited tens of thousands of volunteers. They then randomly split those people into two groups. One group got the actual vaccine. The other was given a placebo injection that contained no medicine, just a saline solution. (Both mRNA vaccines require two equal-sized doses given weeks apart. The Pfizer vaccine shots are supposed to be given three weeks apart, and the Moderna four.)

The trials are called "double-blinded" because neither the volunteers nor the people who gave the shots knew who received the real vaccine and who the saline. Both groups were then monitored for several weeks. Researchers counted new infections for people in each group, as well as the side effects they suffered. In the Pfizer trial, about 20,000 people received the vaccine and the same number a placebo. For Moderna, each trial arm contained about 13,500 people.

The logic behind clinical trials is simple. When we balance two groups this way and give one side a treatment – whatever it may be – and the other a placebo, we can safely assume the treatment is responsible for what happens later, good or bad. Thus, if fewer people get Covid after receiving the vaccine, the vaccine deserves the credit, assuming the trial is run fairly.

By all accounts, the trials were professionally run. Their honesty is not in doubt. So when Pfizer and Moderna announced their amazing findings in November, the world rejoiced. The vaccines seemed to have stopped Covid almost completely.

What almost no one understood at the time was what Pfizer and Moderna *weren't* saying.

Vaccines in general are often the subject of conspiracy theories. These new mRNA Covid vaccines have attracted more than their fair share – that they contain tiny computer chips, can make people infertile, or are even part of a plan to depopulate the planet.

I'm not going to fall into those rabbit holes. I don't even want to spend much time on speculative but more realistic theories about possible long-term harms from the vaccines, such as the risk that they can lead to a dangerous rebound effect in people who later become infected with Covid. Scientists call that possibility antibody dependent enhancement, or ADE. But we don't have much evidence that ADE is a real risk for the Covid vaccines, and I have too much other ground to cover. Focusing on catastrophic but rare possibilities lets pro-vaccine absolutists dismiss other more likely problems.

In fact, the potential risks or questions about efficacy I'm raising are hardly conspiracy theories. *They are visible in the side effect and efficacy data from the vaccine trials themselves.*

They are also visible in the novel biotechnology used to make these vaccines and in their incredibly fast development, as well as the financial incentives that drive drug companies. Remember: governments paid for most Covid vaccine development. Governments buy the vaccines. But for-profit companies make them. Pfizer has already told investors it expects to make about $4 billion in profit in 2021 alone on its vaccine. Meanwhile, the top executives at Moderna and Pfizer's partner BioNTech have made billions of dollars in the last few months, thanks to their soaring stocks. Not millions. Billions. To ask them to remain objective about what they are selling with so much money at stake is to ask the impossible.

The biggest problem with the Covid vaccines is how little evidence we have that their *overall* benefits outweigh their *overall* risks. The question turns out to be much more complicated than whether the vaccines cut the number of Covid infections. That's especially true for people under 50, who face a low risk of serious illness or death from Covid but often suffer severe short-term side effects after being vaccinated.

People over 70 are at higher risk from Covid and appear somewhat less likely to suffer severe side effects from the vaccines. For them, the most important caveat is how well the vaccines will actually protect them.

That question is also more unsettled than vaccine advocates admit.

Understanding why requires a bit of background on how vaccines work. Vaccines prepare our immune systems so they are primed to attack a dangerous virus even *before* we are infected with it. The idea dates back to the 18th century. A British physician named Edward Jenner realized he could deliberately infect people with cowpox, a mild virus, to protect them against smallpox, a deadlier illness. The Covid vaccines use far more complex technology, but they have the same goal.

One crucial step in vaccine development is showing that the vaccines help people make antibodies that will attack the virus. For Covid vaccines, the antibodies target what is called the virus's "spike protein." Those proteins sit on the coronavirus's shell and allow the virus to attach to receptors on the surface of human cells and get inside. Antibodies bind to those spikes, keeping them from attaching to the receptors.

We know the Pfizer and Moderna vaccines help people make those protective antibodies (more on how they do that later). But we also know older people generally make fewer antibodies than younger people. What about the older people who need the *most* protection from Covid, people over 80? The companies didn't disclose anything specific about how people that age responded to their vaccines. Yet those are the people whose immune systems don't respond well to vaccines in general.

(https://www.ncbi.nlm.nih.gov/pmc/articles/PMC1315345/)

In other words, the Covid vaccines — like most vaccines — may work much better in younger people, who are at lower risk from Covid anyway.

Until recently, this risk could only be classified as theoretical. But on March 5 a team of German researchers published their findings from a study that tested how well people over 80 responded to Pfizer's vaccine compared to those under 60.

Unfortunately, the researchers found that vaccines produced a markedly weaker immune response in older people than those under 60. Seventeen days after receiving their second dose, about one in three people over 80 had *no* detectable "neutralizing antibodies" to the coronavirus in their blood – a crucial measure of immunity. Only 1 percent of younger people had no neutralizing antibodies.

(https://www.medrxiv.org/content/10.1101/2021.03.03.21251066v1.full)

Other studies show that the protection the vaccines offer probably peaks between one to four weeks after the second dose and then slowly declines. Thus the researchers were measuring people at what should have been the peak of their vaccine-generated immunity. Yet many people over 80 were still apparently vulnerable to the coronavirus at that point.

Our real-world experience with flu vaccines raises similar concerns. The evidence that influenza vaccines reduce deaths in people over 65 is weak. In fact, a 2020 study that looked at 170 million flu vaccinations in Britain found they appeared to be linked to slightly *higher* rates of deaths and hospitalizations.

(https://pubmed.ncbi.nlm.nih.gov/32120383/)

The Covid vaccines have been given for fewer than four months, so scientists are only beginning to accumulate data on how well they work in the real world. (I will return to this issue in the final section.) What we can say for sure at this point is that the clinical trials did not answer the most important question about the mRNA and all Covid vaccines – whether they actually save lives.

That knowledge gap is no accident. I'm not offering a conspiracy theory, merely stating a fact: Pfizer and Moderna ran their clinical trials in a way that ensured they would *not* have an answer to that question when they asked for permission to sell their vaccines.

This statement runs contrary to most of what you've heard about the vaccines, so let me explain.

Pfizer and Moderna ultimately reported 366 Covid infections in their big trials (counting from one to two weeks after the second shot, when the vaccines become fully effective). Nineteen of the infections occurred in people who received the vaccines. The other 347 occurred in those who got placebo shots.

19 v. 347. Those were the numbers the companies highlighted in November, the numbers that excited the world.

But what no one seemed to understand, then or now, was that those were not hospitalized patients, much less people who needed intensive care or died. They were almost all mild or moderate cases – meaning a positive Covid test along with symptoms such as a cough or low-grade fever.

Serious illness from Covid in the trials was vanishingly rare – not just among people who received the vaccine, but those who got the *placebo*. Out of the more than 13,000 people in the Moderna trial who received the placebo, only nine required hospitalization for Covid. For Pfizer, only nine placebo patients out of 20,000 became what the company defined as "severely" ill, compared to one vaccine recipient. Hospitalizations were rarer still.

The trials also had almost exactly the same number of *deaths* in people who received the placebo or vaccine. No one died of Covid in the Pfizer trial. One Moderna placebo recipient died of Covid, the only patient to die of Covid of all 70,000 people in the two trials. Counting every death that occurred for any reason, or "all-cause mortality," eight people who received the vaccine died, compared to 11 who received the placebo.

Given the size of the trials, that tiny difference offers no evidence to suggest the vaccines either save or cost lives.

Why did so few people die in the trials if Covid has really killed more than 500,000 Americans – 1 out of every 600 people? Because both companies tested their vaccines mostly on healthy people and those under 65. They included only a few elderly people with serious medical conditions, who are the people far more likely to die from Covid than anyone else.

Only 1,700 of the 40,000 participants in the Pfizer trial were over 75. And only half of those received the vaccine. Worse, only Pfizer enrolled only *five* people over 85 in its trial – even though people that age make up one-quarter to one-half of all coronavirus deaths in most countries. For Moderna, the figures are similar.

Detailed data on both the Pfizer and Moderna trials is available in briefing books from the Food & Drug Administration and the European Medicines Agency, Europe's equivalent of the FDA. I will refer to it throughout this booklet.

(https://www.fda.gov/media/144245/download)

(https://www.fda.gov/media/144434/download)

Regulators could have made the companies test the vaccine on more older people.

But they didn't. Instead they focused on making sure the trials were racially diverse. In August, Dr. Fauci encouraged Moderna to enroll more black and Hispanic people. Non-white people were more likely to die of the coronavirus, so they should be properly represented, he said. Trials should "aim to match the burden of disease," Fauci said. "We'd like to do that."

(https://www.cnn.com/world/live-news/coronavirus-pandemic-08-20-20-intl/h_7161d63767b4e937f63049d2d3002d46)

On Sept. 4, Moderna said it would slow its trial slightly to increase non-white enrollment.

Making sure trials are demographically diverse is a worthy goal. Fauci is right that minorities have died from Covid at higher rates than whites (though some of the difference may unfortunately stem from the fact that African-Americans have higher rates of severe obesity and diabetes than whites).

But the difference in death rates between races is tiny in comparison to the difference between older and younger people of any race. People over 80 are *thousands* of times more likely to die of Covid than healthy people under 40. Think of the difference between the risk of flying and driving drunk – very drunk – for a sense of the gap.

Further, the older people the companies did enroll were relatively healthy. Most did not have illnesses like diabetes. But most people who die of Covid have several serious health problems. For example, the Italian National Institute of Health reported in January that two-thirds of people over 70 who died had at least three conditions like high blood pressure, dementia, or other problems. Fewer than 3 percent had no conditions.

(https://www.epicentro.iss.it/en/coronavirus/bollettino/Report-COVID-2019_27_january_2021.pdf)

The importance of this mismatch cannot be overstated. The companies failed to test the vaccine in the "right" people – the people at high risk of dying from Covid. Thus they failed to prove it actually reduced deaths, leaving a tragic hole in our medical and scientific knowledge.

Worse yet, the trials offered some evidence that – as the real-world flu vaccine experience shows and as the German antibody study suggests – the Covid vaccines are less effective in older people. In people over 65, the Moderna vaccine prevented infection 86 percent of the time instead of 94 percent. For the Pfizer vaccine, the rate was 92 percent in older people, compared to 95 percent overall. Those numbers still look solid. But they are in people over 65. No one can know from the trials whether effectiveness decreases further for the extremely elderly.

Could the companies have enrolled more older people and answered the question of whether how well the vaccines worked for them, if regulators had insisted?

Yes. The proof actually comes from clinical trials for other Covid medicines.

In January, Eli Lilly & Co. reported on two studies of its monoclonal antibody treatments for Covid. Unlike vaccines, which boost the body's own immune system, the Lilly treatments attack the virus with antibodies made in laboratories.

Lilly's trials were far smaller than the vaccine trials. But Lilly focused them on high-risk patients, including people in nursing homes. The results were striking.

On Jan. 21, Lilly reported findings from its Blaze-2 clinical trial. It included 340 nursing home residents in the trial. None of the residents who received antibodies died of Covid – compared to *eight* who received a placebo shot. (Remember, only one out of 35,000 people who received the placebo shots in the vaccine trials died of Covid.) In addition, residents given antibodies had an 80 percent lower chance of becoming sick with Covid.

Five days later, Lilly reported equally compelling results from its Blaze-1 trial. The company enrolled more than 1,000 high-risk patients who received either a combination of two antibodies or a placebo. Ten people who received the placebo died, compared to none in people who received the antibodies.

(https://prn.to/3jkoSRv)

(https://bit.ly/3txcvG7)

The Lilly trials prove that enrolling relatively small numbers of high-risk patients can show a treatment makes a big difference in Covid deaths. If they had each enrolled another 3,000 patients over 75, perhaps half of those in nursing homes, Pfizer and Moderna would had have the chance to answer the question of effectiveness once and for all.

Why didn't they?

Not because of cost.

Even if enrolling a few thousand more elderly people had cost the companies tens of millions of dollars, the expense would have been insignificant compared to their potential sales. The United States and Europe are paying about $20 a dose for the vaccines, meaning they have already promised to spend $60 billion on them. Sales to other countries will be tens of billions of dollars more. (By way of comparison, the biggest-selling medicine in the world, an arthritis treatment called Humira, sold about $20 billion worldwide in 2019.)

If money wasn't the problem, what was? One possible reason: enrolling older people might have slowed the trials. And Pfizer and Moderna were racing to be first to market.

After all, vaccines aren't like other medicines. By design, they are only supposed to be given once or twice. A vaccine maker that gets to market a year late may find itself basically shut out.

But there's an even more important reason.

What if the companies had found the vaccines had *not* worked in those elderly patients? What if they had not cut serious illnesses or deaths?

To be clear, that's not necessarily what would have happened. Maybe the vaccines would have worked well in people over 75, just as the Lilly antibodies did. But we don't know. That's why regulators make drug companies run clinical trials – to find out if their drugs work, and what side effects they have.

Scientists and physicians have a term for this: clinical equipoise. The phrase is a fancy way to say, *we're not sure whether this treatment does more harm than good. Better test it.* Equipoise is the opposite of the *do something, anything* mentality some doctors (and patients) have.

But equipoise and business decisions don't always match. Pfizer and Moderna knew they wouldn't need to answer the question of whether their vaccines reduced deaths. As long as the topline data looked impressive, the pressure for approval would be huge. No one would look too hard at what the trials had actually proven – that the vaccines reduced moderate illnesses in people who were at low risk from Covid anyway.

And Pfizer and Moderna were right. The lack of data did not stop regulators from rushing the vaccines ahead. Internal documents from the European Medicines Agency, which regulates drugs and vaccines across Europe, show the pressure that the EMA and FDA faced to approve the vaccines quickly.

The documents are mostly emails that were hacked from the EMA sometime in late November or early December. (On Jan. 25, after previously refusing to do so, the agency confirmed that they were real.)

The pressure began almost as soon as Pfizer announced its initial results on Nov. 9, and only increased in the days that followed. On Nov. 16, Marco Cavaleri, the agency's Head of Health Threats and Vaccines Strategy, told his colleagues the FDA was being "pushed hard by Azar and US GOV." Azar refers to Alex Azar, the Secretary of Health and Human Services, the FDA's parent agency.

Initially, the FDA had told the EMA it did not expect to authorize either vaccine before year-end, giving it a bit more than a month to review the data, the emails show. But the FDA and EMA believed British government intended to move faster, putting pressure on them to do the same.

"They [the British] are going to rush," Cavaleri wrote.

The European regulators faced pressure of their own. Noel Wathion, the deputy director of the European Medicines Agency, told other senior EMA officials in Nov. 19 that falling too far behind the FDA or British regulators to approve the vaccines "may not be easily acceptable." He added, "the political fallout may be too high, even if… [regulators] could defend such a delay in order to make the outcome of the scientific review as robust as possible."

The FDA even asked Pfizer to wait until the end of November to submit its application officially, so it would have a few extra days. But Pfizer refused, applying on Nov. 20 and announcing it had done so – publicly starting the clock on the agency's review. By Nov. 23, the FDA had up moved its timeline to mid-December, giving both its own scientists and outside experts only weeks to review the clinical trial data on the vaccine's safety and efficacy.

But even that timeline wasn't acceptable. By Dec. 1, Donald Trump's chief of staff had already summoned the FDA's commissioner to the White House to explain why the agency hadn't approved at least one, if not both, of the mRNA vaccines.

(https://www.axios.com/fda-chief-called-to-west-wing-0963a1cb-f2c0-4140-b5d9-1441356ada6e.html)

Then, on Dec. 2, the United Kingdom became the first nation in the world to authorize the Pfizer vaccine for sale. Statnews.com, a well-respected Website that covers the drug industry, reported the news this way: "U.K. approves Pfizer's Covid-19 vaccine, putting pressure on FDA."

Big media outlets were equally insistent that the vaccines needed to be approved as quickly as possible. At the time, positive Sars-Cov-2 tests and hospitalizations for Covid were rising, and public health experts predicting a dire winter. "The long darkness before dawn," The New York Times headlined a Nov. 30 article. "With vaccines and a new administration, the pandemic will be tamed. But experts say the coming months 'are going to be just horrible.'"

After an outside committee of experts voted 17-4 on Dec. 10 to recommend the FDA authorize the vaccine for use, the agency had no choice but to act immediately. The next morning, Fri., Dec. 11, then-President Trump tweeted that the agency was "a big, old, slow turtle." Later that day, the Associated Press reported that "a high-ranking White House official told the agency's chief he could face firing if the vaccine was not cleared by day's end."

(https://bit.ly/3pCrGuP)

And indeed, that Friday night, the FDA approved Pfizer's vaccine.

Only it didn't. Not exactly. None of the vaccines now being used in the United States has received full approval. Instead the agency has given all of them what it calls an "Emergency Use Authorization," or EUA. The FDA created this designation in January 2017 to allow the fast sale of medicines during emergencies.

The difference may seem merely a bureaucratic distinction. It isn't. The standard for emergency use is lower than for full approval. The agency requires only that a medicine or vaccine "may be effective" – not that it actually *is*, the regular standard. It requires only that the "known *and potential* [emphasis added] benefits of the product outweigh the known and potential risks," even only slightly.

(https://www.fda.gov/regulatory-information/search-fda-guidance-documents/emergency-use-authorization-medical-products-and-related-authorities)

Given the pressure it faced, the FDA had little choice but to agree the trial results were enough to meet that limbo-stick standard. Exactly one week after Pfizer's authorization, Moderna got its own okay.

Vaccinations began almost immediately, on Dec. 14 for Pfizer's vaccine and a week later for Moderna's. Side effects followed fast.

2

On Dec. 18, Dr. Gregory Michael, a Miami obstetrician, received his first dose of the Pfizer vaccine, becoming among the first people in Florida to get the shot. Three days later, Michael, a healthy 56-year-old, noticed dark red spots all over his hands and feet – a sign his blood wasn't clotting properly.

He went to the emergency room at Mount Sinai Medical Center, an unassuming hospital complex beside the blue waters of Biscayne Bay. There doctors found his platelets – tiny cells that help clot blood – had been destroyed. A normal platelet count is 150,000 to 400,000 platelets per microliter (millionth of a iter) of blood. Gregory's platelet count was zero. Even a small cut could have killed him.

He was immediately hospitalized. For the next two weeks, specialists tried everything they could think of to bring his platelet counts back to normal.

They failed.

On Jan. 3, the blood vessels in Dr. Michael's brain began to bleed uncontrollably. He suffered a hemorrhagic stroke, a painful and terrible death. "Do not let his death be in vain please save more lives by making this information news," his wife Heidi wrote on Facebook two days later. (https://www.facebook.com/heidi.neckelmann/posts/10157817790183977)

Pfizer quickly denied any responsibility for Michael's death.

"We are actively investigating this case, but we don't believe at this time that there is any direct connection to the vaccine," the company told CNN. "There have been no related safety signals identified in our clinical trials... or with the mRNA vaccine platform."

(https://edition.cnn.com/2021/01/06/health/coronavirus-vaccine-doctor-death/index.html)

The statement was not quite true.

Pfizer's big clinical trial had not shown problems with platelets. But a patient had died after suffering thrombocytopenia – the medical term for low platelets – in the *Moderna* trial. (The company and investigators classified the death as unrelated to the vaccine.) Further, rats dosed with other Moderna vaccines had shown worrisome changes in the ability of their blood to clot, according to data Moderna provided to the European Medicines Agency.

Those vaccines were based on the same technology – what Pfizer called the "mRNA platform" – that Pfizer and Moderna used. In fact, because the Moderna vaccines targeted many different viruses, the European regulators wrote that "observed toxicities were not product specific, but rather caused by the immunologic responses towards the translated antigens, and potentially by a contribution of the novel LNP formulation."

That last sentence requires translation.

The Pfizer/BioNTech and Moderna vaccines work differently than older vaccines. Those are usually built directly around the virus, or antigen, that scientists want to defeat. The virions – viral particles – in the vaccines are "inactivated" and cannot replicate themselves. Still, our immune systems will recognize the particles as foreign invaders and respond to them.

The human immune system is incredibly complex. But it has two main defense mechanisms – called "humoral" and "cellular" immunity. Those come out of special cells called B- and T-cells. B-cells fire out antibodies when they come across viral particles in the blood. Those antibodies are the frontline infantry of the immune system. They come in many different shapes. Most are useless against a particular virus. But some randomly may have the right shape to attach to and defeat the viruses. With the help of T-cells, B-cells then learn to produce more of those useful antibodies.

T-cells also play a second role, directly attacking and destroying cells that viruses have infected. They recognize the cells as infected because those infected cells "present" the viral particles to them on their surfaces. This strategy of self-destruction carries its own risks. But if a virus has become entrenched, destroying the cells it has hijacked can be the only way to keep it from overrunning the body.

While our immune systems work to recognize and kill these viral invaders, the viruses themselves frantically invade our cells to make more copies of themselves. Bacteria are living organisms and can replicate themselves if they can find a source of energy. But viruses are nothing more than strands of genetic material – called RNA – inside protective envelopes. They must use our cellular machinery to reproduce.

For this reason, virologists generally do not refer to viruses as alive or dead, but as "replication-competent" or not. But once they do enter a cell, viruses are remarkably good at taking it over to clone themselves. A viral infection becomes a race between the virus's ability to hijack cells and the immune system's ability to destroy it.

Usually, our immune systems win before the virus can do too much damage. But not always, especially in people whose bodies have been weakened by age or other diseases. The immune response itself can also prove harmful, causing inflammation that damages the kidneys, lungs, and other organs. Still, in general, we need a strong response from B- and T-cells to beat back viral invaders. Priming our immune system with vaccines that contain bits of the virus aims to strengthen that response.

But the Pfizer and Moderna vaccines work differently. In a way they are more like coronaviruses themselves. Each vaccine shot contains billions of copies of artificially engineered mRNA – the "m" stands for messenger – each held inside tiny shells of fat called lipid nanoparticles. The shells protect the mRNA strands from our immune systems, which would otherwise destroy them before they reach the cells that are their targets.

Instead, those cells grab the lipid nanoparticles and digest them. Then they break them open, revealing the RNA strands inside. The freed RNA strands go on to hijack cellular machinery just like RNA from real viruses does. Only instead of making a full coronavirus, the RNA delivered in the vaccine tells the cell to make just one part of it – those spike proteins that our antibodies naturally target. Each molecule of injected RNA makes thousands of spike proteins before it degrades. Some escape into the blood and cause B-cells to produce antibodies. Others get stuck on the surface of the cell, where they trigger T-cells to destroy them.

But unlike whole coronaviruses, the spike proteins can't reproduce any further. Once the RNA a person has been given in the vaccine is gone, the body will stop making spike proteins. The "infection" will end once our immune systems destroy the ones it has made. But should the real virus actually infect a vaccinated person, his immune system will be primed and ready to recognize them.

So goes the theory behind mRNA vaccines.

And the theory *works*. The vaccines *do* cause people to make spike proteins. Our immune systems *do* react to those proteins by creating antibodies to them and teaching T-cells to recognize them.

That's the good news.

The bad news is that that's not all the vaccines do.

The idea of using mRNA to trick cells into making proteins has been around for decades. But artificial mRNA strands are very unstable molecules. They have to be kept frozen or they will disintegrate. More importantly, our bodies don't want to be tricked this way.

That's where the lipid nanoparticles come in. Lipid nanoparticles are made up of several different molecules, including cholesterol and polyethylene glycol. They protect the mRNA strands. But they do so at a high price. As soon as they are injected, the nanoparticles provoke their own immune response.

For months, public health experts have sold the idea that the side effects the mRNA vaccines produce are *good,* because they prove our immune systems are working. "The immune system tends to only remember things that hurt somewhat... a bit of pain can be a positive sign that good things are happening. Sometimes you have to earn your immunity," Shane Crotty, a top vaccine scientist at the La Jolla Institute for Immunology, tweeted in November.

(https://twitter.com/profshanecrotty/status/1332425816370683905?lang=en)

In an article in *The Atlantic* in February, writer Katherine Wu detailed the pain her husband suffered after being vaccinated:

> At about 2 a.m. on Thursday morning, I woke to find my husband shivering beside me. For hours. He had been tossing in bed, exhausted but unable to sleep, nursing chills, a fever, and agonizingly sore left arm. His teeth chattered. His forehead was freckled with sweat....

But Wu's story came with a twist:

> And as I lay next to him, I felt an immense sense of relief. All this misery was a sign that the immune cells in his body had been riled up by the second shot of a COVID-19 vaccine, and were well on their way to guarding him from future disease.

(https://www.theatlantic.com/health/archive/2021/02/second-vaccine-side-effects/617892/)

So the story goes. The fevers and chills and nausea are just T- and B-cells attacking the spike proteins we've made – and thus learning to recognize the coronavirus should it ever show up.

One does not need a PhD in virology to recognize the holes in this comforting tale. Effective vaccines against other viruses produce far fewer serious side effects than the mRNA vaccines. Even some other *coronavirus* vaccines produce fewer side effects.

Thus the side effects may be related not to the spike proteins the body is making but to either the mRNA itself or the lipid nanoparticles. No one can seriously consider those side effects a *benefit* of the vaccines – they are off-target problems we must tolerate.

A 2016 paper coauthored by a Moderna founder explained the polyethylene glycol element of the lipid nanoparticles might prove especially dangerous. Repeated intravenous injections with such molecules had been shown to cause "acute hypersensitivity," the authors warned. Both the Pfizer and Moderna vaccines are given as shots in muscle rather than injections directly into the blood, so the risk is lower.

Still, the authors warned mRNA vaccines remained unproven. Because of their risks, they would probably have to be used first as anti-cancer treatments for patients with cancer who lacked other good options (mRNA strands can theoretically help the immune system target cancerous cells just as they help it target viruses). Only then could they be offered to as anti-viral vaccines for healthy people:

> Currently, no mRNA therapeutic is approved for use in humans, and a beneficial safety profile in patients still has to be demonstrated. **A first clinical application will likely not be a prophylactic vaccine**, because the tolerance for side effects is very low for a drug that is injected into healthy individuals.

(https://pubmed.ncbi.nlm.nih.gov/27075952/) (Emphasis added)

But our coronavirus fears turned that equation upside down.

In early 2020, as epidemiologists warned of tens of millions of coronavirus deaths worldwide, the risks of rushing a vaccine seemed small compared to those of the virus. The United States government called its multi-billion dollar effort to jumpstart vaccine development "Warp Speed" – a reference to Star Trek's fantasy that spaceships could travel faster than the speed of light. (The Miriam-Webster dictionary now defines warp speed as "the highest possible.")

Unfortunately, even after we realized the coronavirus was far less dangerous than we'd initially feared, governments rushed vaccines ahead. Normally, drug companies spend years on "preclinical" development, testing potential medicines in laboratories and on animals. Their goal is to choose the best possible candidate before trying it on few healthy volunteers.

Then they spend months or years more reviewing those early human trials and making sure they know everything about possible side effects. Only then do they begin the large "pivotal" clinicals necessary to approve their drugs.

But Pfizer/BioNTech and Moderna compressed that five- to 10-year timeline into months. Moderna started testing its vaccine, called m1273, in humans on March 16, 2020 – barely ten *weeks* after the first reports of the coronavirus emerged from China. BioNTech began its human testing about a month later, in April.

(https://www.cnbc.com/2020/03/16/first-human-trial-for-coronavirus-vaccine-begins-monday-in-the-us.html)

(https://timesofindia.indiatimes.com/world/europe/german-company-begins-testing-possible-vaccine/articleshow/75450971.cms)

Moderna was in such a hurry it did not even finish a proper preclinical study for its vaccine, as European regulators disclosed in their vaccine review. They called the company's work "inadequate for evaluating the repeated dose toxicity of mRNA-1273." They gave the company a pass on the dubious grounds that it had submitted similar preclinical data from other vaccines it was developing.

(https://www.ema.europa.eu/en/documents/assessment-report/covid-19-vaccine-moderna-epar-public-assessment-report_en.pdf)

Moderna's problems should not have come as a surprise to anyone who knew its history. Based in Massachusetts, Moderna was founded in 2010 with the goal of using mRNA technology to make new medicines. The company quickly attracted hundreds of millions of dollars in funding, including a $240 million investment in 2013 from the British drugmaker AstraZeneca.

Stephane Bancel, its chief executive, made bold promises about mRNA treatments. A February 2013 article about Moderna in Boston magazine featured Bancel telling new hires that Moderna would begin testing its drugs in people by the end of that year and might have treatments for previously "undruggable" diseases ready within five years. (It also featured a photo of Bancel in a laboratory wearing a white lab coat, though he is an MBA, not a physician or medical researcher.)

(https://www.bostonmagazine.com/health/2013/02/26/moderna-therapeutics-new-medical-technology/print/)

Moderna could not live up to Bancel's hype. The company didn't put any drugs in human trials in 2013. It was nowhere close to having approved treatments for patients by 2018.

In 2016 and 2017, two devastating articles in StatNews outlined the company's problems. "The company's caustic work environment has for years driven away top talent," Damian Garde wrote in September 2016. "Behind its obsession with secrecy, there are signs Moderna has run into roadblocks with its most ambitious projects."

Garde laid the blame for Moderna's crisis on Bancel:

> Interviews with more than 20 current and former employees and associates suggest Bancel has hampered progress at Moderna because of his ego, his need to assert control and his impatience with the setbacks that are an inevitable part of science...

> Former employees said they felt that Bancel prized the company's ever-increasing valuation... over its science.

(https://www.statnews.com/2016/09/13/moderna-therapeutics-biotech-mrna/)

In a follow-up article in January 2017, Garde focused on the safety issues Moderna faced as it tried to move mRNA treatments from laboratory to the patients. "mRNA is a tricky technology," he wrote. "Several major pharmaceutical companies have tried and abandoned the idea, struggling to get mRNA into cells without triggering nasty side effects."

The side effects increased as patients received more doses of the mRNA drugs. So Moderna had been forced to put aside developing treatments for chronic diseases and instead focus on vaccines – which needed only one or two doses. But in the pre-Covid world, vaccines were considered a backwater of the drug industry, or, as Garde put it – "a less lucrative field that might not justify the company's nearly $5 billion valuation."

Moderna raised another $600 million by selling shares to public investors in 2018. Although the company still didn't have any drugs anywhere near the market, it paid Bancel $59 million that year, making him the highest-paid executive in the biotechnology industry and one of the highest paid in the United States.

Even after it became a public company, Moderna's drug development progressed slowly. By early 2020, it still had not put any of its vaccines into Phase 3 clinical trials, the big studies that must be completed before regulators will approve a drug.

The Covid vaccine changed all that. Throughout 2020, Moderna made sure investors knew how much progress it was making on the vaccine, causing some scientists to question whether it was overhyping its prospects. In May, the dean of the National School of Tropical Medicine called one Moderna announcement "a bunch of opinions in a press release with no data."

(https://abcnews.go.com/US/science-press-release-sudden-rise-vaccine-developer-moderna/story?id=70814887)

Still, investors liked what they heard. By the time Moderna began its pivotal clinical trial for the vaccine on July 27, the company's stock had quadrupled to $80 a share – making billionaires of Bancel and other Moderna executives.

And in the end, of course, the big Phase 3 clinical trial results appeared to vindicate Moderna's hype. 95 percent effectiveness! (Pfizer, which in 2009 pled guilty to a criminal charge and paid a $2.3 billion fine for illegally promoting several drugs for unapproved uses, was more publicly cautious, at least until its Nov. 9 announcement.)

In the excitement, nearly everyone appeared to ignore deeply sobering figures on side effects. The trials made clear neither Pfizer nor Moderna had fully put to rest the concerns that had slowed development of mRNA vaccines for a decade. Their vaccines cause serious side effects in many people, especially after the second shot.

In vaccine trials, drug makers record two kinds of side effects, called solicited and unsolicited events. Solicited events are those that occur shortly after the vaccination itself and are presumed directly related to it, like arm pain or a fever or nausea the day after the shot. Solicited events are generally *temporary* – unpleasant effects that fade as the immune system finishes reacting to the vaccine.

Unsolicited events are more like traditional prescription drug side effects. They can happen days, weeks, or months after vaccinations. They might include anything from a minor rash to a life-threatening infection to a fatal heart attack. They may not be clearly connected to a vaccination – whether the vaccine has caused them is often a medical judgment call.

When the vaccines were being approved, public health experts and journalists downplayed their side effects. They frequently reassured readers that Pfizer and Moderna had found similar rates of problems in people who received the vaccine or the placebo. For example, on Dec. 16, Politico wrote:

> Pfizer's late-stage clinical trial, which enrolled nearly 44,000 people, reported roughly the same number of adverse events in those who received the vaccine — 0.6 percent — compared to 0.5 percent in those who got a placebo.

Those stories were hugely inaccurate.

Pfizer reported in its submission to the FDA that the rates of *unsolicited* serious adverse events were 0.6 percent (roughly 1 in 170) among people given the vaccine and 0.5 percent (1 in 200) among those who received the placebo. The overall figures were 126 to 111, not a big difference considering the trial had almost 20,000 people in each group.

But the media focus on unsolicited events ignored the fact that the rates of *solicited* adverse events were far higher in vaccinated people. Pfizer reported almost 80 percent of people who received the vaccine had pain or swelling where they were injected. Only about 10 percent of placebo patients reported similar problems. The gap worsened as the pain levels increased. About 30 percent of vaccinated people said they had moderate or severe pain, compared to 1 percent of people who received the placebo.

Of course, a sore arm is not life-threatening. And for most people the pain faded within a couple of days. But rates of "systemic" solicited adverse events – like fever, nausea, or diarrhea – were also far higher in people who received the vaccine.

More than 30 percent of people said they had a fever after receiving the vaccine, compared to about 1 percent in the placebo group. 52 percent reported a headache, compared to 24 percent who received placebo. Again the differences increased as symptoms got more severe. Muscle pain, joint pain, diarrhea - a laundry list of symptoms – were all worse in those who received the vaccine.

The Moderna results were similar, only worse. In clinical trials, adverse events are graded on a scale of 1 to 5 – with 1 as minor and 5 as death. Grade 3 events are serious enough to interfere with everyday activities like eating or drinking, like fevers of 102 or 103 degrees. Grade 4 events can be life-threatening.

In other words, Grade 3 and 4 events are not simply a mild fever or needing a few hours rest. For many people, they are more serious than a coronavirus infection would be. In the Moderna trials, about 18 percent reported a fever or other "systemic" problem of Grade 3 or 4, compared to 4 percent who received the placebo.

The huge gap in the rates of solicited adverse events also calls into question the unsolicited events data. People who have already reported side effects early on may not complain again if they have more later.

Even a lot of serious short-term side effects do not necessarily mean the mRNA vaccines are deadly. And no deaths in the clinical trials were definitively linked to the vaccines. But the fact that people in the trials had so many severe adverse events shows they can cause a strong immune reaction – whether because of the lipid nanoparticles, the mRNA itself or some other reason.

Data from both animal and early human studies contained other warning signs, especially about potential blood and cardiovascular problems. European regulators noted that in animals, Moderna's mRNA vaccines reduced lymphocytes – which help fight infection – and increased inflammation. They even caused some precancerous bone marrow changes. The regulators said the changes "were generally reversing" after two weeks. But they did not say the animals had actually returned to normal.

Meanwhile, Pfizer and BioNTech reported their drug caused lymphocytes to drop temporarily in volunteers in an early clinical trial – a sign the vaccine might leave people *more* open to infection in the days after it was given.

(https://www.medrxiv.org/content/10.1101/2020.12.09.20245175v1)

(https://www.medrxiv.org/content/medrxiv/early/2020/12/11/2020.12.09.20245175/F7.large.jpg)

None of these reports by themselves provided reason to reject the vaccines. They *did* provide hints of potential problems that should have been investigated further, or at a minimum tracked once the vaccines were made publicly available. Yet regulators didn't press the companies to run more studies on how the vaccines might damage blood or bone marrow cells.

The animal studies also raised a worrying signal about pregnancy. Both Pfizer and Moderna reported that pregnant rats given their vaccines lost substantially more fetuses than those given a placebo –twice as many for Pfizer, and more than 2.3 times as many for Moderna.

(https://www.ema.europa.eu/en/documents/assessment-report/comirnaty-epar-public-assessment-report_en.pdf)

Those were the *only* studies the companies conducted on pregnant animals. And they specifically excluded pregnant women from their trials. Again, though, regulators did not ask the companies to run more tests on pregnant animals to see if the rat fetal deaths were real or a fluke.

At this point, we simply don't know if the vaccines might be dangerous to fetuses. And pregnant women are stuck without clear guidance about whether to be vaccinated. In a sign of the tension around the issue, one of eight members of a committee that advises Israel's government about vaccinations quit on March 17 because it would not advise against vaccinating pregnant women or at the least warn them about potential dangers.

(https://twitter.com/SelaReport/status/1372538035556995072)

(https://www.mako.co.il/news-lifestyle/2021_q1/Article-84361e349e14871026.htm) – in Hebrew.

But pregnant women aren't the only ones waiting for clarity on the safety of the Covid vaccines. After well over 100 million doses worldwide, we still do not know how often they cause severe side effects, much less deaths.

Some points are clear, though.

As the clinical trial data suggested, the Covid vaccines cause serious and unpleasant side effects in many people. Both the United States and Europe have systems allowing healthcare workers to file reports if see someone have a medical problem after receiving a vaccine. Patients can also file reports directly. The United States system, called VAERS, includes details from the reports themselves, though not the identity of patients. The European system, EUDRA, offers only a broad overview of reports.

Both systems have received far more reports of side effects after Covid vaccine shots than other vaccines. By mid-March, VAERS had received more than 30,000 reports of side effects from Covid vaccines – as many as all other vaccines combined during the last year.

The gap is even larger for reports of serious side effects or deaths. With about 110 million doses of mRNA vaccines given in the United States, the VAERS system had received more than 1,800 death reports, the CDC reported on March 16. In comparison, it received about 20 reports of deaths out of 180 million flu vaccinations in the last two flu seasons.

(https://www.cdc.gov/coronavirus/2019-ncov/vaccines/safety/adverse-events.html)

Based on the number of reports received, people are more than 150 times as likely to die after receiving a Covid shot than the flu vaccine. But that difference *underestimates* the real ratio of death reports per vaccination, because people must receive two shots of the mRNA vaccines to be fully vaccinated. Fewer than 40 million people had received two doses in mid-March, meaning that death reports were roughly 500 times as likely to come in following Covid vaccinations.

Some deaths occurred almost immediately and may have resulted from severe allergic shock, or anaphylaxis. Others occurred days later and were related to cardiovascular problems such as heart attacks or blood problems such as thrombocytopenia, the illness that killed Dr. Gregory Michael. These are exactly the areas that the animal trials highlighted as potential concerns.

Dozens of miscarriages have also been reported to both VAERS and the European side effect database. Miscarriages in early pregnancy are not uncommon. But the reports included several deaths of late second or third-trimester fetuses, which are rare. In one particularly disturbing case, a woman reported having pain just hours after receiving her second dose of the Pfizer vaccine. She miscarried the next day. (VAERS report 0930196).

Vaccine advocates downplay the significance of the side effect databases. With tens of millions of people being vaccinated, some will by chance become very sick or even die shortly afterwards, they argue. After all, at least 5,000 Americans die every day, and the number rises to 9,000 in the winter –

even excluding Covid deaths. Reports to VAERS do not prove that the vaccinations caused the problems, merely that the problems followed the shots.

Many vaccine evangelists go further. They dismiss the reports and discourage reporting on them at all. In February, Vice magazine wrote that "VAERS, a database of reports of vaccine side effects, is being abused by people trying to sow fear."

In reality, without long-term clinical trial data, the side effect reports are the best and arguably the only way to pick up potential problems with the vaccines. And Gregory Miller's case is far from unique. The database includes many reports of deaths and serious injuries in relatively young people who had no previous problems and died shortly after receiving the vaccine – like VAERS report 1006662-1, of a 51-year-old- woman in Texas:

> Patient had 2nd vaccine, went home, and started "cramping" in all of her muscles. It became bad enough that she was taken to a local ED [emergency department] where she then started coughing up blood, required intubation and about 6 hours later, died.

Or 1037027-1, a woman in Utah:

> She had pain in the injection site... and then Tuesday she got worse with nausea and some fever. By Wednesday she was complaining that she could not pee... At 0600 Thursday morning she woke us up and said she needed to go to the hospital... [She] became incoherent... her liver function was all wrong and they started to look for a hospital that could transplant a liver. She was air evade [sic] about 0930 to Medical center and just over 30 hours later she was dead. There is a pending autopsy. She was a healthy 39 year old mother.

Maybe these deaths were mere coincidences. Maybe one or both of these women would have died anyway. Maybe other similar reports are coincidences too. But at the least they would appear to be worthy of serious investigation. Instead the CDC dismisses them with the blanket statement that it has found "no evidence that vaccination contributed to patient deaths."

The irony here is that most states classify *any* death within 30 or 60 days of a positive COVID test as being caused by the virus, even in cases where the death is obviously not linked – like someone shot to death weeks after having had a positive test with no other symptoms. But with vaccines, public health experts try to downplay any possible connections between vaccinations and deaths. And social media companies are actively suppressing posts and videos that raise the issue.

In contrast, European regulators have taken side effects reports more seriously, at least for the AstraZeneca vaccine. In the wake of unusual cases in which people under 50 became ill or died from a combination of blood clots and very low platelet counts, Germany and other European countries suspended use of the vaccine in mid-March. A physician who had led a group investigating cases in

Norway reported that they had resulted from a hyperactive immune response the vaccine had produced. "There is no other thing than the vaccine that can explain that," Dr. Pal Andre Holme said.

https://bit.ly/3qVfSo5) – in Norwegian.

AstraZeneca's vaccine does not contain mRNA, like the Pfizer and Moderna vaccines. But it is also not a traditional vaccine. Instead it uses a cold virus to inject DNA into cells, where the DNA is converted into RNA. The RNA causes those cells to produce coronavirus spike proteins, as the Pfizer and Moderna shots do. In other words, like the mRNA vaccines, it is a novel vaccine that works by hijacking our cells.

And the reports about the AstraZeneca vaccine are similar to some of the most serious reports in the US VAERS database for the Pfizer and Moderna vaccines, including thrombocytopenia (low platelets) and blood clots. In the European safety database, where the number of reports for Pfizer's vaccine can be directly compared to AstraZeneca's, the Pfizer vaccine has had far *more* side effect reports – about 102,000 as of mid-March, compared to 55,000 for AstraZeneca's. It has also more than four times as many death reports and cardiac death reports, 957 and 276 for Pfizer compared to 198 and 63 for AstraZeneca. (The two vaccines have been given a similar number of times in Europe, although exact figures are unavailable. The Moderna vaccine is far less common in Europe.)

Yet European countries have focused their scrutiny on the AstraZeneca vaccine. Even so, they have faced huge pushback from vaccine advocates. "Europe's Vaccine Suspension May Be Driven as Much by Politics as Science," the New York Times wrote, in a story focused almost exclusively on the potential harm of slowing vaccinations rather than the actual cases that had led countries to be wary.

On March 18, following an emergency meeting, the European Medicines Agency said that the AstraZeneca vaccine "may be associated with very rare cases of blood clots associated with thrombocytopenia." Still, the agency said the overall benefits of the vaccine "continue to outweigh the side effects."

One major problem that regulators face is that the clotting risks appear to vary widely by age, with younger people at greater risk – the opposite of the risk of the coronavirus. The EMA reported that the excess risk was confined to people under 55, where it at least 17 very serious cases, including deaths, had been reported over a period when it would have expected only about two cases. But in older people, no excess cases were reported.

As Europe struggles publicly to weigh side effects and benefits of the Covid vaccines, American media outlets and health authorities have generally dismissed them.

One American news outlet has run a comprehensive report on Covid vaccine side effects. It began:

> Like many others, Eunjin Kim felt like she'd been hit with an instant case of influenza after getting her second shot of the Moderna COVID-19 vaccine. "I was laying there with a down comforter and with the electric blanket and still shivering," Kim said.
>
> Carissa Spencer didn't have to wait for her second shot of the Pfizer vaccine to feel like something wasn't right. She had swelling that moved

down the right side of her body. "I was extremely nervous, it wasn't very attractive at all," Spencer said.

The story even mentioned the miscarriage issue, pointing to a woman who had reported suffering a miscarriage after being vaccinated.

Which outlet ran this hard-hitting investigation? The Washington Post? The New York Times?

Try KUTV – a local television station in Salt Lake City. It did the reporting that major national outlets have not. (https://kutv.com/news/coronavirus/covid-19-vaccine-side-effects-deaths-the-lack-of-information-on-how-where-to-report)

Even when the Times choked out an article about the potential link between the vaccines and thrombocytopenia in early February, the paper downplayed it. Its headline ran "A Few Covid Vaccine Recipients Developed a Rare Blood Disorder. A link to the vaccines is not certain…"

(https://www.nytimes.com/2021/02/08/health/immune-thrombocytopenia-covid-vaccine-blood.html)

The skeptical attitude is especially striking because last year, the Times, Washington Post, and CNN linked Covid to an alphabet of ailments. Those included strokes in young people, deadly post-infection inflammation in children, and even "Covid toe."

(https://www.cnn.com/2020/04/22/health/strokes-coronavirus-young-adults/index.html)

(https://www.washingtonpost.com/health/2020/05/21/misc-c-kawasaki-coronavirus-young-adults/0

(https://www.nytimes.com/2020/05/01/health/coronavirus-covid-toe.html)

Maybe the worst example of this credulity came in April 2020, when the Washington Post claimed

> Doctors also are reporting bizarre, unsettling cases that don't seem to follow any of the textbooks they've trained on…. Asymptomatic pregnant women suddenly in cardiac arrest. Patients who by all conventional measures seem to have mild disease deteriorating within minutes and dying at home.

(https://www.washingtonpost.com/health/2020/04/22/coronavirus-blood-clots/)

To put it nicely, time has not been kind to that story.

Yet the same news outlets that credulously reported Covid's potential dangers have largely refused to acknowledge the vaccine can possibly do harm, even as side effects reports pile up.

Worse, just as they've done with masks, they have ignored any scientific studies or data from before March 2020 that might raise concerns. Moderna's troubled past? Gone. Papers on the risks of lipid nanoparticles? Memory-holed.

Nothing can be allowed to raise questions about the vaccines, because only the vaccines will lead us out of the mess of social distancing, empty schools, and shuttered businesses. Only the vaccines will help the millions of Americans who are afraid to leave their homes, much less shop or see friends, after a year of media fearmongering.

Only the vaccines are the answer. Only the vaccines are 100 percent effective.

Yes, supposedly serious media outlets such as MSNBC and public health authorities such as the Los Angeles County Department of Health have claimed with a straight face that the mRNA and other vaccines are "100 percent" effective at ending COVID hospitalizations and deaths.

(https://twitter.com/MSNBC/status/1373130197336227841)

100 percent effective. As in they never fail.

If only.

3

The mRNA vaccinations started in December. Since then, countries have given close to 200 million doses of the Pfizer and Moderna shots – mainly to older people.

That's enough people and enough time to begin calculating how well the vaccines work in the real world, as opposed to the carefully selected participants in the clinical trials. Scientists from several countries have recently done just that, posting research comparing groups of people who have been vaccinated with those who have not.

Different scientists have looked at different outcomes, including infections, hospitalizations, serious cases, and deaths. Independent researchers are also examining the national-level data out of Israel, which has had the most aggressive vaccination campaign of any country. It vaccinated nearly everyone over 70 by late January – almost two months ago.

While the results differ from country to country and researcher to researcher, they broadly form a consistent pattern, one suggesting the Pfizer and Moderna vaccines provide protection – but not as much as the 95 percent the clinical trials suggested, much less the "100 percent" figure that places like MSNBC claim.

Before looking at the details of the results from Israel and elsewhere, it's crucial to understand that researchers generally base their estimates for how well vaccines work on the "fully vaccinated" population. They define that group as people who are at least a week past the second dose of the mRNA vaccines – but no more than three or four weeks, because that's all the data we now have.

Judging vaccines then will put them in the best possible light. That period is when vaccine-fueled antibodies peak, giving people maximum protection. The overall protective effect of the vaccines will inevitably be lower than that peak figure – perhaps much lower. While some vaccines, like those for measles, can offer protection for decades, at this point we have no idea how long vaccine protection will last against the coronavirus.

In fact, Moderna and Pfizer themselves now suggest the vaccines may need to be given every year. In that case, many people are enduring serious post-vaccine side effects for just a few months of protection.

Another important fact in looking at how well the vaccines work: Covid infections have fallen almost everywhere in the world since January, both in countries that have vaccinated and those that have not.

The receding epidemic is great news. But it also means simply focusing on what happens to the vaccinated population in countries like Israel or the United Kingdom can be deceiving. Researchers must adjust those figures for what's happening in the unvaccinated population as well.

To take a simple example: Suppose 100 residents at a nursing home are vaccinated. 100 others are not. In the week before vaccination, 10 of the to-be-vaccinated residents and 10 of the unvaccinated became infected. By the fifth week after vaccination, only one of the vaccinated residents becomes infected. Great! The vaccine seems to offer 90 percent protection.

But what if the unvaccinated residents have also suffered only one infection in that fifth week? They too have seen a 90 percent decline. The vaccine isn't offering any extra protection. The coronavirus has just faded away for everyone.

In the real world, this math is far more complicated. People keep shifting from the unvaccinated to the vaccinated group as the shots continue. An even trickier facet of this shift is that people who are vaccinated *later* have less time "at risk" after being vaccinated than those who got the shot earlier. Announcing millions of people have been fully vaccinated but "only" a few thousand have become infected —as the Israeli government has done — makes the vaccine seem more effective than it is. Many of those vaccinated people have been vaccinated for only a few days, not months.

Also, researchers need to adjust for different risk factors, especially age. But even after making those adjustments, they can't be sure the vaccinated and unvaccinated populations had the same baseline risk. Maybe people who choose to get vaccinated early are more worried about their health and more careful than those who aren't — the same issue that confounds flu vaccine data. Or maybe getting vaccinated makes people feel safe, so they begin to take more risks. In that case, the risky behavior might undercut the effect of the vaccine.

Researchers have developed ways to try to account for these differences, by matching groups of vaccinated and unvaccinated people as evenly as possible, and adjusting for age and other known risks. Still, every after-the-fact adjustment can increase errors.

And many researchers feel clear pressure to paint the most positive picture possible – especially in Israel, where an election will be held on March 23 and the government has staked its future on vaccines. In early February, Eran Segal, an Israeli computer scientist who has advised the government on vaccines, wrote that "the magic has started."

At the time, Israel had far more hospitalized patients and daily Covid deaths than it had when its vaccinations had started in December. To get around this unpleasant truth, Segal and other analysts noted that people over 60, who were more likely to be vaccinated, made up a *relatively* smaller proportion of deaths and hospitalizations than they had before, *even though their absolute numbers had risen sharply since vaccinations began.* As evidence went, this was remarkably weak – but media outlets parroted the claim.

Fortunately, we now have studies with data from other countries too. Danish researchers published the most important on March 9, looking at infection rates in health-care workers and nursing home residents in Denmark. They were among the first people in that country to be vaccinated. Nearly every resident received at least one shot of the Pfizer mRNA vaccine. And the Danish health-care system is nationalized, so researchers had a comprehensive database about what had happened afterwards.

The researchers found the vaccine was about 90 percent effective in the workers a week or more after the second dose. But the rest of the news was less positive. In the nursing home residents – who were 84 years old on average and thus needed the protection far more – the vaccine was only 64 percent effective after the second dose.

Worse, both residents and healthcare workers actually had a much *higher* risk of infection for the two weeks after their first dose. In the residents, the risk increased 40 percent. In the workers, it more than doubled.

(https://www.medrxiv.org/content/10.1101/2021.03.08.21252200v1)

A British paper offered similar results. It showed that the Pfizer vaccine *increased* the risk of Covid by almost 20 percent in the first 10 days after vaccination – and 40 percent in people over 80 who received it first.

(http://medrxiv.org/content/10.1101/2021.03.01.21252652v1)

Probably not coincidentally, nursing homes saw waves of infections as vaccinations ramped up in December and January. "Denmark sees surging COVID-19 infection rate in nursing homes," the Chinese news service Xinhua reported on Jan. 4.

(http://www.xinhuanet.com/english/2021-01/04/c_139641397.htm)

The Danes were not alone. Similar outbreaks occurred in nursing homes all over Europe and North America. One Dutch home reported that 22 of its 106 residents had died in the weeks after vaccinations began. "With the start of vaccinations we expected that the infections would decrease, but that did not happen and we are very upset," a director of the home's parent agency said.

(https://www.rtvutrecht.nl/nieuws/2139404/de-eerste-coronaprik-was-gezet-en-toen-kwam-toch-nog-de-uitbraak-we-zijn-er-erg-ontdaan-over.html)

The worst carnage took place in Britain – the first country to approve the Pfizer vaccine and the most aggressive country outside Israel to vaccinate. On February 1, Dr. Martin Vernon, the former National Clinical Director for Britain's National Health Service, tweeted an urgent warning:

> One month into the care [nursing] home vaccination programme [in Britain], I am deeply concerned to be seeing covid-19 infection outbreaks among first dose vaccinated residents within, and beyond 21 days of vaccination. Are any other clinicians seeing this happening?

https://twitter.com/runnermandoc/status/1356337026757492738

Dr. Vernon was right to be worried. Across Britain, deaths during the winter epidemic peaked almost five weeks after mass vaccination campaigns began in earnest. During a ten-day period in late January, Britain averaged more than 1,200 deaths per day.

That figure is the equivalent of 6,000 deaths a day in the United States, and the worst stretch for any big country since the beginning of the epidemic. Britain has now surpassed Italy as the major industrialized nation with the most coranavirus deaths per-capita.

Israel saw a similar pattern. Deaths peaked in late January, about a month after the vaccinations began. Now other countries are seeing the same trend. Chile began mass vaccinations in early February, for example. Its neighbor Argentina moved much more slowly. As of mid-March, 41 percent of Chileans had received at least one vaccine dose, compared to only 6 percent of Argentinians. That's two in five people on one side of the border, versus one in *16* on the other.

But over the same period, cases have risen 40 percent in Chile. Deaths are up about 15 percent. Meanwhile cases have fallen nearly 15 percent in Argentina and deaths dropped 30 percent.

Beyond the possibility that the vaccines temporarily suppress the immune system, another possibility is that the *act* of vaccinating by itself leads to more infections. Nursing homes that have isolated residents for nearly a year open their doors to vaccinating nurses and medical staff. Elderly people who have largely stayed home go to mass clinics.

The good news is the bump in risk appears to be temporary. The second dose produces a spike in antibodies and a decrease in the risk of infections and serious cases. Positive tests, serious cases, and deaths in Israel and Britain have all declined significantly since their January peak.

The Danish paper is probably the best benchmark, since it appears to have the least political bias. Again, it put the reduction in infections at 64 percent in nursing home residents and 90 percent in healthcare workers, who are younger. One independent researcher looking at Israeli data estimated the overall reduction in deaths at 65 to 75 percent once people are fully vaccinated.

The same British paper that a 20 percent rise in short-term infections after the first dose showed 83 percent protection two weeks after the second dose. Another British paper found a 85 percent reduction in health-care workers. (https://papers.ssrn.com/sol3/papers.cfm?abstract_id=3790399)

Other scientists have estimated even higher figures – as high as 95 to 99 percent for some Israeli researchers. For example, Pfizer claimed on Thursday, March 11, that data from Israel shows its vaccine prevents up to 97 percent of severe cases of coronavirus.

(https://www.jpost.com/health-science/coronavirus-pfizer-vaccine-97-percent-effective-against-severe-cases-661700)

Again, though, the researchers claiming these very high rates of protection generally do not seem to have adjusted for the fact that infections in people who were not vaccinated have also been declining. And they are hard to square with the fact that almost 20 percent of February deaths in Israel came in people who had received both vaccine doses.

Still, the vaccines *do* appear to provide good protection in younger people and at least decent protection even in elderly people once they become fully vaccinated. But there are four big caveats.

First and most importantly, much of the world had a sharp rise in cases and deaths in December and January followed by a plunge in February and March. The pattern held both in countries that vaccinated heavily and early, like Britain and Israel, and those that didn't, like Germany and Canada. So whatever good vaccinations have done on a national level has so far been marginal at best – and is further undone by the fact that the countries that vaccinated early had such sharp spikes in January.

Second, Israeli data show that a small but significant number of older people, between 5 and 10 percent, do not become fully vaccinated. Most of those people receive the first dose but not the second, possibly because they cannot tolerate the side effects of the first dose. They clearly remain at significant risk from Covid. Deaths in people who had received only one dose accounted for almost 40 percent of all Covid deaths in Israel in January and 25 percent in February. So looking only at the "fully vaccinated" substantially overstates the effectiveness of the vaccine.

(https://www.ynet.co.il/news/article/B13FB1TMO#autoplay)

(https://datadashboard.health.gov.il/COVID-19/general)

Third, we don't know yet how long the peak protection will last, so we don't know yet how much of the gains are undone by the apparent short-term increase in risk after the first dose.

Finally, we don't know how many people are suffering serious side effects, so we can't compare those harms to the benefits.

With so many uncertainties, we simply do not know at this point how much the Covid vaccines – both the mRNA and other vaccines – will reduce Covid deaths in either the short- or long-term.

Worse, we cannot even begin to guess whether the vaccines will reduce not just Covid deaths but "all-cause mortality" – overall deaths in people who receive them. All-cause mortality is a high bar to meet, but some drugs do, notably the cholesterol-lowering medicines called statins.

Yet governments did not allow these uncertainties to stop them from embarking on a campaign to vaccinate the world's entire population.

As I promised near the beginning of this booklet, I have mostly avoided the "black swan" concerns that anti-vaccine advocates have raised – that Covid vaccines may cause infertility or make Covid more dangerous to people who are infected after being vaccinated, a process called antibody dependent enhancement.

Those appear to be extremely unlikely.

But I do want to raise one other issue – that vaccines might make Covid more dangerous to unvaccinated people – since scientists have demonstrated it is a real-world risk with at least one other vaccine. In 2015, researchers showed that vaccines for Marek's disease, a herpes virus that causes cancer in chickens, had caused the disease to become much more dangerous to unvaccinated chickens.

As the study's authors explained:

> We show experimentally that immunization of chickens against Marek's disease virus enhances the fitness of more virulent strains... Our data show that anti-disease vaccines that **do not prevent transmission** can create conditions that promote the emergence of pathogen strains that cause **more severe disease** [emphases added] in unvaccinated hosts.

(https://journals.plos.org/plosbiology/article/info:doi/10.1371/journal.pbio.1002198)

Chicken farms worldwide began to inoculate their flocks against Marek's in the 1970s. Since then, Marek's disease has mutated from a slow-moving virus that leaves chickens partially paralyzed but does not always kill them into a pathogen that quickly kills nearly every chicken it infects.

The researchers speculated the change was driven by the fact that the Marek's vaccine was "leaky." It protected vaccinated chickens but did not stop them from shedding the virus. A leaky vaccine might theoretically allow vaccinated chickens to spread increasingly dangerous strains of the virus – which otherwise could kill them – to unvaccinated chickens. In experiments, the authors confirmed the theory.

"Previously a hot strain was so nasty, it wiped itself out," the study's lead author told PBS. "Now you keep its host alive with a vaccine, then it can transmit and spread in the world."

https://www.pbs.org/newshour/science/tthis-chicken-vaccine-makes-virus-dangerous

Of course, chickens aren't people. And most human vaccines, like those for measles, don't have this problem. That's because they are "perfect" or "sterilizing." They offer full immunity to almost everyone who receives them.

But as the researchers pointed out, vaccines for influenza and malaria are leaky. "Our concern here, primarily and foremost, is whether this is going to happen with any of the vaccines that we give to people," a molecular biologist told PBS.

If it is not obvious by now, Covid vaccines are leaky. They do not offer complete protection and the Centers for Disease Control has already warned that "vaccinated people could potentially still get COVID-19 and spread it to others."

(https://www.cdc.gov/coronavirus/2019-ncov/more/fully-vaccinated-people.html)

None of this means that a Marek's disease scenario for Covid is even a remote possibility, merely that it is a theoretical risk – one that vaccine advocates will never mention.

In many ways, the Covid vaccines – especially the mRNAs – have become a real-world Rorschach test.

Vaccine advocates see a scientific leap forward that may work not just against the coronavirus but influenza, other viruses, and even cancer. Just as the terrible injuries of wartime led to advances in surgery, the pressure of the Covid epidemic led companies and governments to work together. They introduced these new vaccines far faster than would have otherwise been possible. Even if some kinks need to be worked out, the mRNA hypothesis has now been shown to work in the most dramatic possible way.

But to vaccine skeptics – anti-vaxxers –the mRNA vaccines are just another in a long line of overhyped vaccines. They are far more dangerous than the scientific community admits and have potentially catastrophic long-term risks. The speed of their development is cause for alarm, not celebration. In the long run, they may cause infertility, devastating brain diseases, or the emergence of devastating new variants of the coronavirus. By the time we know the truth, it will be too late.

As is usually the case in these dogmatic battles, the truth is likely somewhere in the middle. Both sides are so focused on their own gospel that they have failed to see the vaccines for what they really are – a new technology that carries both promise and risk.

The mRNA vaccines clearly can reduce the risk of coronavirus infections. In that most basic sense, they work. And so far we have no evidence to support any of the more apocalyptic predictions of the vaccine skeptics.

But it is equally clear that for many young and middle-aged people, the mRNA vaccines have side effects that are worse than a coronavirus infection would be. The cases of rare but serious blood disorders that have dogged the AstraZeneca vaccine are visible in the side effect reports for the mRNA vaccines too. At the same time, we cannot say for certain how much the vaccines directly help the older people who are really at risk.

Ultimately, the vaccines face the same problem that has dogged every other public health "intervention" for the coronavirus since last March. The virus is far more dangerous to old and unhealthy people than anyone else. But neither the media nor health experts nor regulators will admit that reality. Instead, they are trying to force hugely intrusive "solutions" on billions of people who are at very low risk to protect a much smaller number at higher risk.

This issue is particularly acute in the case of the vaccines since they essentially weren't even tested on older people, while their side effects are worse in younger people. And the questions of personal and parental choice that masks and lockdowns raise pale in comparison to those raised by vaccine mandates or quasi-mandates.

Make no mistake, regulators failed at every point in the development of these vaccines – the preclinical work, the major clinical trials, and the approval process. Then again, they had little choice. Dr. Moncef Slaoui, who oversaw Operation Warp Speed, told the Times that the United States government had realized that "what was very important was to be a full, active partner in the development and the manufacturing of the vaccine. And to do so very early."

How could the FDA or EMA possibly have stood up to that pressure? A few extra weeks of preclinical development might have given us more information about the vaccines' pregnancy risks and other rare but serious side effects. A few thousand extra older people in the trials would have answered once and for all the question of whether the vaccines save lives.

But those questions were never answered. Now they may never be. Weirdly, even the concerns about the AstraZeneca vaccine have not touched the mRNA vaccines. It's not just the people who have been cowering at home for the last year who are desperate to declare the vaccines successful and move on.

Many people who understand the real risks of Covid feel the same. They just want to get on with their lives and they view the vaccine as the way out. In the coming months, the pressure to be vaccinated is only going to increase. Even raising the basic data-driven issues I have discussed in this booklet causes massive backlash, as I have learned since January.

But that doesn't make them any less real.

Made in the USA
Monee, IL
23 April 2021